THE DENTAL PRACTICE BREAKTHROUGH

Finally Win over Patients by Conquering the 5 Devastating Marketing Mistakes That Are Costing YOU Big

JACKIE ULASEWICH

COPYRIGHT

TABLE OF CONTENTS

TABLE OF CONTENTS

FOREWARD

In *The Dental Practice Breakthrough*, I will walk you step by step through the five major marketing mistakes that are costing you and your practice big. You'll learn to recognize the difference between a gimmick and a genuine marketing strategy, how to enhance your online presence, and how to build lasting relationships with your patients that make them feel valued beyond their semi-annual cleaning appointments. All of these strategies are necessary to retain your current patients, expand your practice, and stay competitive with both the new dentist down the street and the pervasive corporate practices that seem to dominate the industry.

These strategies are applicable regardless of the size of your practice or years in dentistry. Dentists who are opening their first practice, those who need to build business in order to bring in an associate and eventually retire, or those who have been in practice for years but simply don't have the marketing know-how to make a well-needed change—it is necessary for each of these practices to create a digital presence that will allow them to succeed as much as (if not more than) corporate dentistry and their neighboring dentist. The online landscape is oversaturated, competition is fierce, and there are marketing agencies that promise their clients the world but deliver unoriginal, templated materials that do NOT help them stand out above the rest.

There is much more to marketing than bringing in new patients and being rated #1 on Google.

ABOUT JACKIE ULASEWICH

How did I get here? When I was fresh out of college and seeking jobs in marketing and business development, I was contacted by a dental laboratory for an interview. What I knew about dentistry at that time could have filled a thimble; I wasn't even sure what a dental laboratory did. To prepare for the interview, I visited a few local practices and asked them to help me understand how a lab fit into the big picture. The information was helpful, but if I wanted to be hired, I would need to stand out from the scores of other college graduates that would be interviewed.

One of the practices I met with happened to have a lab box from the very laboratory that I would be interviewing with and graciously allowed me to keep it. I prepared for my interview: In one impression tray I wrote my first name, on the other tray I wrote my last, and on the lab script I wrote, "I wanted to leave a lasting impression." After being interviewed by a panel of five people, I slid the lab box across the table. This calculated risk landed me my first job in the dental industry.

Once I was hired, I became a student again. I met with anyone I could who was willing to share their knowledge; I learned their industry, I learned their lingo, I learned their processes, and I learned their challenges. I spent ten years observing and doing market research in hundreds of practices across the United States and quickly became an expert in my field. With my newfound knowledge, I was able to assess the needs and struggles of individual practices as well as the fallibilities of the marketing industry itself.

The importance of helping others has been ingrained in me since I was a little girl, so bettering an industry that I was passionate about seemed like a logical choice. I observed the marketing industry become more corporate and more concerned with their own needs, not those of their clients. Starting a business that was passionate about helping, considerate of the solo practitioner, and excited about implementing marketing strategies that work was just what the doctor ordered. Just as I did for my job interview, I wanted to run a business where I could find a "lab box" for each of my clients; something personable, well-planned, and customized to make them stand out among the rest.

At that point, I made the decision to move away from corporate marketing. As a small business owner, I can relate to your trials and triumphs. I care about each of our clients—not just the bottom line. So many agencies focus on checking off boxes on a list, not on the specific needs of each individual client. When marketing is done on this mass scale, companies fail to provide their clients with the level of service they deserve. This parallels what is happening in the world of corporate dentistry; some corporations have a huge marketing budget and have their eyes on their profits, not what is right for their patients.

Starting my own business opened my eyes to specific struggles that small business owners have. Suddenly, I found myself in charge of billing, bookkeeping, accounting—all things I did not have the know–how or time for. Much as I hesitated, I opted to hire an accountant to handle my books. Your situation is likely similar: you went to school to become a dentist, yet as a business owner you are responsible for hiring, billing, managing—none of which dental school prepared you for. Hiring a huge marketing company may be tempting; you already have so much on your plate. But if your marketing company isn't customizing their approach, integrating all your digital campaigns, and helping you enhance your relationships outside your practice, then you are simply wasting your money. Worse, you are not serving the needs of your patients.

My experience in the field has helped me create philosophies and practices that work for both my business and those of my clients:

- I take a comprehensive, customized approach to my business; every strategy is carefully crafted for each client.

- I focus on enhancing relationships with existing patients, not just bringing in new business. If your bucket is filling up but there are holes in the bottom, then you are wasting your efforts.

- I integrate marketing solutions by using multiple channels and making sure the channels work seamlessly together. I use Facebook, blog posts, websites, remarketing, paid ads and emails working together to create a complete strategy.

- I create fun, relatable, and unique marketing tools that stand out in a sea of repetitive, templated, and uninspiring materials.

The Dental Practice Breakthrough will change the way you market your practice. You will learn the common mistakes that keep your practice from being the best it can be, but—best of all—you will learn how to remedy those mistakes and make your practice one that patients will brag about.

fewer posts about dentures, implants, and dental problems that few 20-somethings have to deal with. Whatever the content of your posts, the feelings and images you want to have associated with your practice must be present to make your patients know that you—not a mass marketing agency—have taken the time to communicate with them.

CHAPTER TWO
Mistake #2: Limiting Your Focus to Bringing in New Patients and Google Rankings

It makes sense that bringing in new patients will help you grow your practice and create increased profits, which is why marketing companies make these promises: "We will get you new patients," "Your phone won't stop ringing," "Get new patients NOW!" The problem with this approach is that it is myopic and fails to consider the big picture.

One approach to bringing in new patients is to emphasize site rankings on Google. Google uses an algorithm to determine the popularity of each site. Essentially, the more popular the site, the higher up on the search results list it goes. Google rankings are generated by SEO, or Search Engine Optimization. SEO writing *alone* is tricky; too few keywords and your post gets overlooked, too many and it registers as spam and gets both overlooked *and* flagged. When you combine the writing complications with all of the other factors at play, emphasizing and only focusing on SEO for the purpose of ranking is simply too risky. Marketing companies convince doctors of the urgency to rank higher, completely ignoring the quality of the site, usefulness to the target audience, and templated content that could be considered to be spam. Do you only focus on fixing the patient's cracked tooth with a crown, veneer, or bonding and never look at what truly caused the issue? No! Because it fails to consider the big picture and understanding if the patient is grinding or if the teeth are out of alignment. This is the same as focusing all of your marketing on bringing in new patients or being on Google's top twenty results. Ranking is important, but to put all of your efforts into ranking is not the right strategy. What good is a page one ranking if your reviews are largely negative? What good is a page one ranking if potential patients click your link only to find an outdated website that makes them continue scrolling? Our philosophy is to focus on the big picture, which is why we don't limit our efforts to only rankings and new patients.

Marketing companies that limit their focus to bringing in new patients are ignoring other vital facets of a solid marketing strategy, including your current patients. Filling a bucket that has holes in the bottom is a futile task; what good are new patients if your current patients are disappearing out the back door? When you ignore your current patients, you are more likely to lose them to practices that are more conveniently located, or worse, to the omnipresent corporate practices.

For the most successful marketing strategy, it is imperative that you look inside your practice as well as out. With the right information and a little attention, your current patients can be your best marketing tool. Patients who feel valued are more likely to remain loyal, and loyal patients are more likely to refer your practice to the new patients that you seek.

Instead of focusing on the rank of your website, focus on making connections with the people who are giving you their business *right now*. Remind them on a regular basis that they are part of *your* practice's family and that you are part of *their* lives well beyond their semi-annual appointments. There is no doubt websites are an important marketing tool, but the best way to get web traffic is through word-of-mouth and other strategic marketing campaigns, not a templated site that lacks personality.

CHAPTER THREE
Mistake #3: Using Multiple Vendors for Your Marketing Campaigns

An effective marketing campaign is completely comprehensive and focuses on the 3 R's—reputation, relationships, and retention (which will be addressed in section two). For genuine success, you should be firing on all cylinders, looking at the entire picture instead of putting all of your effort into one or two channels such as Google pay–per–click and email. Your marketing strategy will be ineffective and disjointed if you:

- Have a website but do not update your blog posts regularly

- Send emails but do not redirect patients to your blog, which lives on your website

- Send emails but do not redirect patients to like or follow your social networking sites

- Have a Facebook, Instagram, Twitter, or SnapChat account but only post once or twice a month

- Use review sites that do not get sufficient traffic

When you work with multiple marketing vendors and don't

treat marketing as a part of your dental team, then none of your campaigns are working together. At first glance, it may be appealing to find the cheapest web designer, cheapest Facebook guru, and the cheapest writer for your emails (who, more often than not, is you). The problem with this approach is that none of the information is integrated and synthesized; all of your marketing channels should feed off of one another. For example:

- An email campaign should invite people to read your most recent blog, schedule an appointment, and follow you on social networking.

- Your website, where potential patients view your blog and schedule appointments, directs patients to social networking sites and solicits reviews.

- Your social networking sites provide opportunities for your patients to like or follow your practice, leave reviews where they'll be seen, and invites them to click a link to read your latest blog, schedule appointments, or sign up to receive emails from your office.

When one of your patients refers a friend or family member to your practice, their first instinct will be to check out your digital profile. If your email works with your website, which works with your social networking sites, which works with your online reviews, potential patients will be able to know what you and your practice are about in a matter of seconds. They will know that your content has been customized, they will see your favorable reviews, they will observe your interactions with patients on sites like Facebook and Twitter, and they will learn through pictures and other engaging posts that you value your staff, your patients, and your community. Every resource you use must work in tandem to give your prospective patients the incentive to become a current patient.

Another tool that ties all of your marketing efforts together is Remarketing. Remarketing is a way for your practice to stay in front of prospective and current patients once they leave your website by displaying your practice branding on the subsequent sites they visit. Whether they're booking a trip on Travelocity, making a dinner reservation through OpenTable, or seeing what's just dropped on Netflix, your practice branding will appear as a reminder that they've recently been on your site. Need a clear picture of the impact that remarketing can have when it is integrated with other campaigns?

Imagine that your patient, Betty, is drinking wine with her favorite neighbors. Her friend, Jane, begins to complain about her smile, so Betty mentions your practice. Jane picks up her smartphone and finds your website, but while cruising your site their other friend, John, elicits laughter from the entire group with a classic joke, so

Jane sets her phone down to rejoin conversation. Clearly, Jane had every intention of reading more about you and your practice, but she got distracted, as most of us do on a regular basis. Good thing you have a remarketing campaign, because over the next few days, weeks, and months to come, Jane will see an ad for your practice when she is browsing the web or checking her newsfeed on Facebook. This simple integration of remarketing to your website visitors reminds Jane that her good friend, Betty, recently referenced the best dentist in town, so she picks up the phone to call and request an appointment.

You need to approach your marketing just like the marketing department of a large corporation would; you must have a clear objective in mind and know which strategies will help you meet your objectives. Many of the practices I speak with on a regular basis are working with multiple vendors for their marketing, each of whom has their own objective, agenda, and individual style. There is no big–picture strategy, instead they are running one or two campaigns that are not designed to work together.

True success lies in consistently using multiple integrated strategies that allow you to meet your objectives. When you deploy a Facebook campaign that does not align with your email campaign, spend thousands on a website that doesn't include a remarketing code or isn't kept fresh with new, customized content, or send emails that don't include a link to your website or social networking pages, you are wasting your money. Nine out of ten dentists that My Dental Agency speak to say that we are one of the only agencies who consider the big picture. There is a reason why you should have a marketing partner versus a marketing vendor.

DIGITAL MARKETING CASE STUDY

The Challenge

We Fixed Something They Didn't Know Was Broken

Dental practices are in the smile repair and beautification business. What we've found is that the bigger challenge for dental practices is knowing how best to showcase their expertise in a way that helps them stand out and effectively reaches their core patient base through digital marketing. We think some practices fear embracing digital marketing and even the lighter side of dentistry, making it difficult to capitalize on the education they have to share. Perhaps that's understandable. It must be a bit traumatic when you run an office that is not exactly the destination at the top of anyone's list!

The Strategy

How to Digitally Market Your Way into a Prospective Patient's Heart

Patients need to trust their dentist and dentists need to build lasting relationships with their patients. A dentist's sharpest tools are education and personality. That is, useful information about treatment options to support informed decisions, to strengthen relationships, and ultimately to spread the word about their cool office and compassionate dentistry. Our client wanted to enhance the relationship with their current patients and reach them outside of the practice and didn't know where to start. So our team got together and started brainstorming and we thought... where better to demonstrate these than on social media platforms and email campaigns?

So we asked our client to let us shake up their digital marketing strategy over a nine month period to see how it enhanced relationships, increased interest in additional treatment options and help broaden their practice awareness and in just as little as four months we saw tremendous results.

They were beyond impressed to say the least. Well, all we can say is: Numbers Don't Lie!

The Results

Growth of their Facebook page resulting in enhanced relationships with current patients & increased visibility in the South Tampa Bay area

800% increase in page likes in 4 months.

Facebook Reviews and Ratings

of reviews were generated after we started managing their page. No reviews were solicited, these actions were solely from organic growth and exposure.

Page Impressions

Impressions are the total number of times activity related to a page is seen by people (current and prospective patients) on Facebook, whether they see it organically, virally or via a paid advertisement.

Over four consecutive months that count was exactly:

2,222. *Like, wow!*

Monthly Pageviews

Pageviews are the number of people who have viewed a Facebook page, current and prospective patients.

They had **599** views in 4 months

Increased website traffic/Increased page views on website

One of our goals for social media and email campaigns are to send patients and prospective patients to the website to view services, read blogs, contact the practice and of course request an appointment.

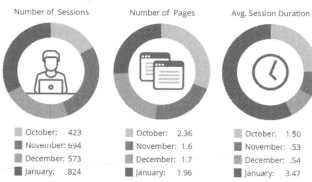

Number of Sessions	Number of Pages	Avg. Session Duration
October: 423	October: 2.36	October: 1.50
November: 694	November: 1.6	November: .53
December: 573	December: 1.7	December: .54
January: 824	January: 1.96	January: 3.47

Email open and click rates

6% click rate on links to request an appointment

161 total clicks (for appointment requests, checking out their site and Facebook page and blog)

Needless to say, this client was grinning from ear to ear after four months — as are all of their new and existing patients!

The moral to the story? Embrace Digital Marketing, it's the lifeblood of every business and profession.

CHAPTER FOUR
Mistake #4: Failing to Use the Unique Personality of Your Practice in Your Marketing

Mistake number four points directly back to mistake number one—using a cookie cutter instead of a custom approach to your marketing. Your personality is the one thing you have to offer that no one else does, and it should be present in everything from your website, to emails, blog posts, your Facebook page, and so on.

It's important for you to identify the personality of your practice. Are you whimsical and silly? Is your office more professional and conservative? Are you tech savvy and a bit on the nerdy side? Do you love anything that has to do with music and use that as a way to connect with patients? Whatever your practice personality, it should permeate your marketing efforts. The impression you give in person should be consistent with the impression you give online. When a new patient sees an ad on Facebook, looks at your newsfeed, or visits your website, they should feel that they already know you; when they finally visit your office, they should know exactly what to expect based on the personality you projected in your marketing materials. This consistency builds trust with your patients—prospective and current—and helps to ease anxiety about visiting your office. Your goal should be to start a positive relationship with your patients before they have a chance to step through your door. If you're using any of the following in the materials you present to your patients, you're already starting off on the wrong foot:

- Stock images from the web (the perfect family with their smiling children, stunning hygienist working with an adorable white–haired patient, gloved hands holding instruments up to a faceless–but–charming smile)

- Copied and pasted blurbs and articles from a library of content (From the ADA archives or the proprietary platforms of marketing agencies, you see it again and again and again and again)

- Generic, unbranded content (repetitive or not, it could work on the site of Dentist A, Dentist B, or Dentist C because it is completely devoid of personalization)

Another consideration to make when determining what image you want to project is your target audience. Are you are trying to attract a younger, hipster, or even millennial demographic? Having a high–tech office in a prime location is a good start, but if your website is outdated, your Facebook newsfeed is full of boring articles, and you have no reviews on Google, then you are not going to connect with a young, upwardly mobile patient base. Similarly, if your patients are predominantly retirees, then limiting your social networking to SnapChat or another platform that is unfamiliar to older generations will result in missing out on *their* business.

Achieving the perfect balance of an authentic personality that appeals to your target demographic is vital to your marketing strategy. Companies who dump weak, repetitive content in your lap and expect you to deploy that information on your own time are not considering your needs. Do you know the ideal time to post on Facebook? Do you know how to login to the dashboard of your website and upload a blog? Do you have time to figure out either of those things? You want to *remove* one of the many hats you wear, not *add* to them. An effective marketing strategy will incorporate your personality and take care of the details that you're far too busy for, allowing you to focus on your patients.

CHAPTER FIVE
Mistake #5: Using Mundane and Boring Marketing That Appeals to No One

I spent many years in the dental industry, all the time witnessing dental practices playing it safe, using the same, boring, mundane marketing. I rarely—if ever—came across a piece of marketing that truly lended itself to the practice and made me feel connected. Why is that? At the time, it was the industry norm to conform.

These days, the digital landscape is noisy. The Internet is littered with ads, trying to gain our attention at every turn. In this saturated climate, it is essential that you do something that is fun, attention–grabbing, and shows who you are. There is no reason that dentistry can't be fun!

I have made it my mission to bring a little life into dental marketing. Consumers have more options than ever, and they want to feel connected to the people they chose to do business with; they want to know that there is a real person at the other end of the advertisement. Why not give them what they are looking for by using your personality combined with some levity? So many people fear going to the dentist and they need reassurance; they're also smart enough to see through the canned garbage of poor marketing. If we can use your marketing campaign to put them at ease and make them feel like they are a part of your dental family, then we will have achieved something great.

To engage your patients, avoid overwhelming them with statistics and sales pitches. They enjoy seeing what they won't see on other sites, such as:

- Photos of you and your staff at celebrations and community events; these show your patients that you know how to have fun, that you enjoy being with people, and that you value making contributions to the community.

- The benefits of purchasing new equipment or bringing in an associate dentist; what matters to your patients is what these changes can do to improve their quality of life.

- Fun contests with easy giveaways; this could include trivia, scavenger hunts on your site, or even a call for patients to share awkward adolescent smile pictures on your social networking feed. People like winning, even if the prize is only glory or a travel toothbrush, toothpaste, and floss set.

- Share memes and gifs that validate but bring levity to the idea that many people, no matter how old, fear going to the dentist; allow your patients to see that you understand where they're coming from *and* that you have a sense of humor.

SECTION TWO
Why Digital Marketing is Important

I began my marketing career in a more traditional world and understand the challenges very well. When I attended college, digital marketing wasn't a part of the curriculum. Even when I graduated and entered my first position, traditional marketing —specifically postcards, television, billboards, and radio—was king. Like many dentists feel today, I was hesitant to make the shift into digital marketing. However, once I saw the countless ways I would be able to track the results and how cost effective these campaigns can be, I was sold.

With online technology, you can optimize your marketing campaigns in real time and evaluate their cost effectiveness. Hesitance to make the leap into the digital realm is understandable, especially if you do not consider yourself to be technologically savvy. The truth is, the marketing world is evolving; if you wish to stay relevant and stay in front of your patients, then digital is a must. Need cold, hard facts to convince you?

• Thirty–four percent of patients say their choice of dentist is greatly influenced by the quality of the practice's website.

- A staggering number of people (about 94%) use their mobile phones to search for local information, including looking for a dentist.

- Reviews are extremely important; 70% of your patients say that reading online reviews influenced their choice of dentist, even if the practice had been referred by a friend or family member.

Of the 7.2 billion people on earth, 3 billion have Internet access and 2.1 billion are active on social media (Link Humans), so it's reasonable that your potential patients expect to find you online. The Pew Research Center shows that 90% of adults ages eighteen to twenty–nine use social media and that 52% of online adults use *two or more* social media sites (Pick). Even if your target demographic is an older generation, statistics indicate that people from the ages of fifty to seventy–five are active online using search engines such as Google and social networking sites like Facebook. In a 2015 study of the online habits of baby boomers, DMN3 found that 91% of the people surveyed used one or more social networking sites, with Facebook in the lead at 84.9 % (Lockard). To dismiss older generations as "old school" is to underestimate what they can bring to your practice. Like any other age group, boomers *need* your services and *want* to find a practice that they connect with.

CHAPTER SIX
The 3 R's: Reputation

Having a positive online reputation is the foundation for all of our marketing efforts. Even when a trusted friend or family member refers a new dentist, that individual is going to do their online research well before they schedule an appointment. The reputation you project is essential to marketing your business, whatever campaign you might run.

If you are focusing on bringing new patients on board, be prepared for them to do a thorough search online. They will look at your website, see what kind of reviews you've been given, check out your Facebook page to see how many followers and posts you have, and see if your practice is listed in local directories. You may be active in your community by using postcard campaigns or other media to attract new patients, which is effective as long as you also have an online strategy. Having a website—even one that is stellar—is not enough. It's only a small piece of the puzzle.

Consider your online reputation: What digital channels are you using? What are your patients seeing when they search for your practice? The most likely sources are:

- Google reviews

- Facebook page and reviews

- Yelp (Yep! Yelp is even important for Dentists)

- HealthGrades

- Yahoo, Bing, and so on…

How is your practice presented on all of those sites? Do you have an up–to–date profile that includes a current photo, practice description, updated hours, and address? If these aren't part of your digital presence, how do potential patients perceive you? Are you projecting an image that would make them choose your practice over your competitors?

Your reputation isn't about being listed on these high–traffic websites. To get someone to make the jump from scanning your page to sitting in your chair, you must have a good number of recently posted positive reviews on as many of these sites as possible. Being represented by a couple of reviews on one or two sites is insufficient; current, frequent, expansive, and positive reviews will help you achieve the success that you deserve.

Of course, it is inevitable that your practice will eventually get a negative review. Often times, these reviews are simple misunderstandings or completely out of your control (such as problems with insurance coverage), which is why it is vital to keep your positive reviews rolling in. When you know that a patient has had a positive experience, ask them to share it with the online world. When good reviews far outnumber the bad, the former rise to the top and the latter get pushed to the bottom.

Maintaining a positive online reputation is essential to the growth of your business. Without it, the casual web browser will have no incentive to contact your office to make that first appointment.

CHAPTER SEVEN
The 3 R's: Relationships

Building strong relationships with your current patient base is key to your marketing success—after all, they are the people who have put you on the map and are helping you maintain your practice *right now*. As mentioned in Section One, many marketing campaigns make the mistake of focusing on new business while they ignore their existing patients. If you are not capitalizing on the people you already see, then you are wasting your efforts and losing money.

We know that it's difficult to build a lasting relationship with your patients when you only see them twice a year (and sometimes less). That is exactly why it is crucial to the success of your practice to stay in front of them year-round using all the available online resources. Being active on social networking sites and utilizing custom emails gives you the opportunity to do two things:

1. Enhance your efforts outside of the four walls of your practice, and

2. Build lasting relationships with your patients

This is not accomplished by posting once-a-month templated content on Facebook, sending cookie-cutter emails that don't address the needs of the individuals who you are reaching out to, or using the same, bland web copy that looks just like every other practice's site. Because marketing is not what you went to school for, you can often overlook the fact that the persona you present online is *identical* to hundreds of other professionals. So how is that helping you build your relationships with patients?

Consider how you feel when you see content—both online and off—that is clearly templated. You know the marketing pieces I'm referring to: they use stock photography, non–personalized messages, and are sometimes poorly branded. Now consider how you would feel as a consumer if you saw this material while searching for a medical doctor for your child, parent, or even yourself? Would seeing the same copy posted again and again on websites and Facebook feeds instill faith in you about their practice? Even if you were referred by a friend or family member, this would give you pause. Your patients are reacting the same way if your marketing materials aren't giving them the confidence to commit to you as their dentist.

To make patients know that you want to connect with them, genuine, customized marketing is necessary. What you post should make your patients proud to be associated with your practice and encourage them to pass your information along to their friends and family. It should be content that they'd be proud to forward and share with their online community.

Being active online is a start, but if you want to create patient loyalty, you need to have a strategy. Your strategy should always include these things:

1. Education on a level that is relatable and not too technical for your patients to understand

2. Information that explains the benefits and not just the features of your services

3. Personalization—online and off—that allows you to build lasting relationships with your patients

Here's an example of how your online presence can connect you with your patients:

Say that in the last year, you've treatment planned fifty patients for a specific service—such as implants, whitening, or Invisalign—and they haven't moved forward with treatment. In most cases, you only connect with those faces one or twice that year. Think about the power of using a customized email campaign to connect with them multiple times after they leave your building, educating, reminding, and incentivizing them to follow through with their treatment.

Another example is connecting with patients via Facebook. As your patients scroll through their newsfeed and see what is going on in your office, they are likely to react or comment on your post. When they do that, there is a possibility that their friends and family are going to see that interaction. In utilizing social networking sites, not only are you deepening your relationships with your current patients, you're also getting in front of potential patients.

When your online efforts remind patients of you on a regular basis, they are more likely to talk about your practice to friends and family, leave you a review, and do such things as "check in" on Facebook while at your office. All of these are ways for you to increase your online presence, get in front of prospective patients, and make your current patients know that they matter to you every day of the year—not just when they're in your office.

CHAPTER EIGHT
The 3 R's: Retention

There is a reason all of this is so important: if you use our proven marketing strategies, you'll be engaging with your patients consistently throughout the year—much more frequently than their semi-annual appointments. When you do this, you achieve amazing results:

- Your patients become extremely loyal and less likely to leave you for your competitors.

- Your patients will be engaged with you online, consistently sharing your content with others.

- You will create social proof; when prospective patients find you online, a large percentage of them will see that their friends and family have "liked" and engaged with your practice.

- You will establish a constant, ongoing, positive patient experience both inside and outside of your practice.

You and your staff do an excellent job making your patients feel important when they're in your office; those efforts should not end when they walk out your door. When you create patient loyalty, they are more likely to accept treatment plans and talk about you to their friends and family. This results in an organic referral campaign.

Focusing On the Three R's

Focusing on the 3 R's is what it takes to take your marketing campaign from fair to first-rate. These are the steps that you need to take in order to beat the corporate dental practices and to distinguish your practice from your competition around the corner.

Herein Lies the Rub

How can you avoid the five mistakes that are detrimental to your marketing effort, practice the three R's, *and* give your patients the attention that they deserve? By finding a marketing company that you trust and can rely upon; one that has your best interest at heart.

In an ideal world, your dental training would have included business education. In a perfect world, you would have time to serve your patients, meet the needs of your staff, balance the budget, return all of your messages, have a personal life, hang out with your family, and market your business. You can do *anything*, but you can't do *everything*, so to alleviate some of the pressures that come with being a successful business owner, you must find a marketing company that is willing to work with you closely, able to understand the "big picture," and be focused *not just* on quantity, but quality.

The Dentist Guy to Breakthrough

SECTION THREE
Remarketing, Social Media & Your Website

In this section we will go more in depth on some of the most important points covered in the first two sections.

Get ready to learn more about remarketing and how to engage your patients on Facebook and Twitter with a social media strategy that works. We will discuss how to minimize the impact of the inevitable negative reviews and how to implement an email campaign that will get results. You will learn the importance of having a "good" website and how a blog can help build rapport with patients. Finally, we discuss reputation management and the steps you can take to assure that yours is top-notch.

CHAPTER NINE
Remarketing to Extend Your Reach

Have you ever been searching online for a new pair of running shoes, or maybe a new car mechanic, and while you are browsing on those sites, either the dog barks or someone knocks on your door? Or, maybe you see you have a new message on Facebook—and before you know it, you clicked out of newbalance.com and on to something new? We all have, probably multiple times a day.

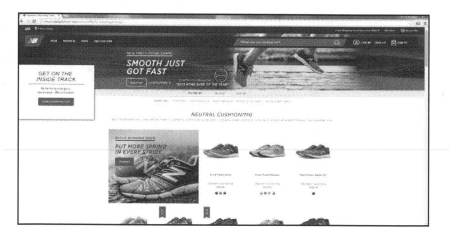

So what happens to that new pair of running shoes? If you're like most people you've probably forgotten about them. What does this have to do with remarketing? Everything!

On average 95–98% of visitors are leaving your website without taking action.

That means most of your visitors come to your site and don't call your office to make an appointment or fill out your new patient form. Why? Because they got distracted, or maybe they are doing research and comparing various different offices, or they're just not ready to decide if they want to get their teeth whitened or have that cracked tooth fixed.

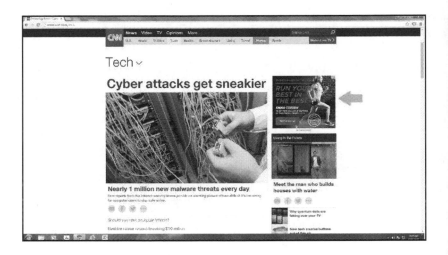

But back to our running shoes example. Fast–forward three days and you're reading an article on cnn.com and you see the same pair of running shoes in an ad on the right hand side. You notice the display ad on the side and it reminds you that you meant to make that purchase and never did. So what do you do? That's right; you click on the link and make the purchase. That is remarketing!

At this point you are probably thinking one of two things, "Wow that is really neat and I want to learn more," or, "How can this help my dental practice and what are some numbers to support this marketing effort?" Well, let's dive a little deeper to help you better understand.

Let's start with why remarketing is so successful, along with some results, and then we can discuss the process of how you can launch these campaigns.

INEXPENSIVE — you can start with as little as $50/month.

CONVERSION — remarketing customers are 70% more likely to convert compared to someone who has not been remarketed to.

SUCCESS RATE — 49% of individuals visit a site 2–4 times before they actually convert.

COMPETITION — most consumers visit multiple sites before making a decision. If you are the only dentist in your area not remarketing, you are leaving money on the table.

Just in case you need additional convincing on how dental remarketing can help your practice, here are a couple more reasons. *(For additional information go to www.mydentalagency. com/dental-marketing-services/remarketing.)*

Visitors will continue to see your brand and messaging for free, which helps you bring awareness to your practice.

Another positive aspect of a remarketing campaign is, although you will only pay when visitors click on your ads, we know the individuals seeing your ads already have interest in your practice because they visited your website. This means if they take action and click on the ad they must really be interested!

So how does remarketing work? It's actually pretty simple. When a visitor lands on your website a cookie is stored in their browser that is later used to uniquely identify them. As that same visitor browses other websites in the days, weeks and months following, that cookie containing the visitor's unique identifier is used to determine where they've been previously, allowing the ad networks to serve them remarketing ads for those previously visited websites.

There are a couple requirements:

1. You must have a website

2. You must have a minimum of 20–100 unique visitors per month

I implore you to consider remarketing for your practice. It may seem optional now, but I can assure you it won't be. Don't wait until all of your competitors have caught on!

Recent studies have shown that visitors who were re-marketed to were 70% more likely to take action compared to those who weren't.

CHAPTER TEN
How to Engage with Patients Online Using Facebook and Twitter

No longer is it a matter of should, but must. The need to leverage social media to retain and gain patients is indisputable. With communication having undergone such a transformation in recent years, the only way to remain relevant, and therefore successful, as a dental practice is to join the conversation via social media.

By nurturing a relationship with your target audience, you can cultivate patient growth within your practice. If you provide useful information to patients and potential patients, you can become approachable, which is so central to creating a positive patient experience online using popular social media platforms such as Facebook and Twitter.

A Social Media Strategy That Works

Despite the array of social media platforms, your best strategy is to conscientiously maintain a couple well. In other words, "kill it" on Facebook and Twitter. This goes in particular for Facebook. In September 2014, 71% of the U.S. online population had a Facebook account, according to a Pew Research Center social networking fact sheet. Facebook also provides access to a storehouse of invaluable demographic data, such as potential patients living within a 3–to–5–mile radius from your dental practice.

5 Facebook Best Practices to Know

1. Build your following. Don't spin your wheels posting to a Facebook page with only a few followers. Develop that fan base first. Here's how:

   - Ask patients in an email campaign to "like" your Facebook page.

   - Grab current patients' attention about your Facebook page with compelling office signage.

   - Motivate your team to share posts from your practice's page and even request a few patients per day to "like" the page or review a recent visit.

   - Purchase a Facebook ad. Unlike traditional forms of advertising with a blind reach, Facebook ads are precise. Set an ad budget at $1 or $2 per day to build your following. Cost–effective and super–targeted, you can start by creating a customized audience of existing patients by using their email or phone numbers and then devising an ad requesting a page "like."

2. The 80/20 rule: 80% of the posts should present fun, relevant, engaging content, while 20% should focus on your

services and practice. No one wants to be sold to all of the time. As part of the content comprising 80% of your statuses, post pictures of your staff, actual patient photos (with the patient's written consent), photos from charity events and holiday parties, and short, fun, "Did You Know?" tips and facts. Audiences also respond better to images that you've taken instead of stock photos. The goal is to showcase what humanizes your practice and make your practice relatable.

When you are posting the service-related content making up the other 20% of your statuses you can direct people to your website to request appointments and learn more about your services, show them before and after photos, and talk about new patient or service specials.

"Liking" your page is not authorization for your patient to receive an around-the-clock infomercial. It means someone is showing an interest so provide information of value to the patient or potential patient. Social media is not all about you.

3. Dig deeper.

Facebook offers its own analytics. Use Facebook's "Audience Insights" feature to see who is engaging with your posts for demographic detail such as gender, age, and location. You can also discern which day(s) and time of day in general are best for posting. This will provide an understanding of who is engaging on your page, when they are engaging, and what they are finding interesting. Informed with that level of detail, you can customize future posts.

4. Although it is helping your business, Facebook is a business, too.

    Facebook wants you to post content that it thinks your friends and followers want to see. It is also very much a pay–to–play platform. It doesn't cost much, but boosting a post here and there helps you reach your audience and beyond. You can spend $2 or $3 per post and reach a much broader audience.

5. Social media is no "set it and forget it" business–building strategy.

    If someone comments on a post, reply to them within 24 hours. Not only does replying show the patient you care, but it also shows potential patients who may be looking at your page that you take the time to engage. Social media etiquette also dictates that you extend gratitude when someone posts a review.

Top 3 Twitter Tips

Although a great channel to impact a broad audience, Twitter is a veritable fire hose of information. Still, it is a viable forum to tweet relevant events or news and links to your practice's website and blogs, to follow local people and companies, and to engage with the community. With this baseline of 140 characters, you should:

1. Tweet multiple times a day.

2. Make use of hashtags that give your tweets keywords so your information can be easily found.

3. Use shortened URLs such as goo.gl, ow.ly, or bit.ly. These are not lengthy, and as a result are more readable, as well as allow for tracking of how many people clicked your link.

Some of the same principles of Facebook apply to Twitter, such as this important one: *No one wants to be sold to all of the time.*

Today's patients need to feel a sense of comfortability. They are not selecting a dentist based on sheer geography; rather, they are choosing ones they believe they can trust because they feel they know them. Maintain a robust, genuine presence on key social media platforms, and both your practice and your patients can reap generous rewards.

This article originally appeared in the August/2016 issue of the Academy of General Dentistry's AGD Impact magazine.

CHAPTER ELEVEN
How to Handle Negative Reviews

Reviews are one of the most useful tools that the Internet has to offer. Anyone with a smartphone can use Angie's List, Consumer Reports, Google, or more before deciding when and how to spend their money. When you're a business or dental practice on the bad end of a review, however, the World Wide Web can seem small and unfriendly.

A negative review doesn't have to destroy your digital presence, though. With a few smart tricks, you can even use a zero–star rating to demonstrate your loyalties to your patients.

Positively Proactive

The best thing to do to avoid negative reviews is to be proactive. Before patients leave your office, ask them about their experience. If they were pleased, suggest that they leave a review. If they weren't, handle it right then and there to let them know they are valued.

Also, use an *email campaign* to solicit reviews from your regulars—who, let's face it, wouldn't be regulars if they weren't happy with you. Make sure that your positive reviews far outweigh your negative reviews. That way, the negative reviews won't stand out so much or hold a lot of weight. *(For additional information go to www.mydentalagency.com/dental-marketing-services/email-marketing.)*

Stop Negativity in Its Tracks

The occasional negative review is inevitable. Whether it's due to a miscommunication or something completely out of your control, unhappy patients leave negative reviews to gain a sense of control over their situation. When you do receive a negative review, address it immediately and publicly so others know you take your reputation seriously.

Suppose a new patient was asked to wait longer than he expected. The anonymity of online reviews allows him to exaggerate to his heart's content and claim that your office has no time management and does not value your patients' time. This is an opportunity to make that person feel that he matters, as a little validation goes a long way.

Respond to that patient with an apology, thank him for giving you an opportunity to improve your practice, and offer to have an office manager call to discuss his disappointment. Not only is this a best practice, but also anyone who reads that review will see that your practice prioritizes the needs of your patients.

Bottom Line

Even when referred by a friend or family member, consumers use your Internet presence to determine if your practice is right for them. Managing your website, email, and *social networking* pages might be technologically tricky and time consuming, but doing so is well worth the effort. If negative reviews are addressed quickly, and positive reviews keep rolling in, you're bound to be "liked" in more ways than one. *(For additional information go to www.mydentalagency.com/dental-marketing-services/dentists-social-media.)*

This article originally appeared in 2016 in Dentistry Today.

CHAPTER TWELVE
Strategies for Successful Email Campaigns

Social media has revolutionized the marketing industry, but as great a tool it is for business, it still has some limitations. Even if you use platforms such as Facebook, Twitter, Instagram, etc., there's a chance that your patients may miss one of your posts or only get a certain amount of information. When you want to reach them directly and go more in-depth about something noteworthy at your practice, sending an email just might be the way to go.

Reaching your patients via email is still the best way for your office to send them customized messages that target their specific needs and interests. Consider how different your patients are from one another: You've got those who come in twice a year for cleanings and dental exams; you have patients that you may see once a year—if you're lucky—and you have people with more extensive treatment needs who visit the office every couple of months. Your email campaign can be just as diverse as the people who sit in your chair, and there are several strategies that you can employ to make the most of the messages you send to them.

Get to the Point

Like you, your patients are busy, so make your emails easy to read. A lengthy form letter can appear overwhelming and is likely to be deleted immediately. Instead, use subheadings, numbers and bullet points to break the content up into easily absorbable chunks. Your patients will be more likely to take the time to read something that can be skimmed and then revisited when they have more time.

Have Some Fun

Keep the tone of your email messaging light. An email that is too technical won't be relatable to people outside your field. And don't be afraid to experiment with subject lines and the type of content you feature. Consider including some of the following:

- Pictures of staff functions such as office birthday parties or other celebrations ("Doctor Joseph celebrates five years at her Main Street location!")

- Dental trivia from movies or television shows ("What was the name of Jerry's dentist on 'Seinfeld'?")

- Oral health and hygiene tips ("10 Acidic Foods to Avoid to Protect Your Enamel")

- Information about events happening in your community (health fairs, charity events, etc.)

- Staff member biographies ("Meet Dental Hygienist Joe Smith")

Point Out the Perks

The emails that sell products and services still should be written to be meaningful to your patients. For example:

- Don't just tell your patients that you purchased a new intraoral scanner for your practice; explain how that equipment will ultimately improve their dental health and make the time they spend in your office more enjoyable.

- Don't simply send an email about the new associate joining the practice; let your patients know if this dentist offers a special skillset or if she or he will be available during times that you are not. Without those explanations, your patients will have no idea why they should care about your new hire.

Engage Your Patients

Use an email campaign to give your patients multiple ways to stay connected to you. Include hyperlinks to the social networking sites that you use and encourage them to "like" or "follow" your practice on social media and leave favorable reviews. Drive more traffic to your website by including hyper-links to your blog, and make scheduling an appointment convenient for your patients by using a "request an appointment" option. All of these strategies provide additional opportunities for you to reach out and make connections with your patients.

Be Consistent in Your Email Outreach

The ultimate goal of using an email campaign is to make sure your patients are reminded of your practice beyond their occasional office visits. There is no need to overwhelm them with weekly messages, but your emails should be sent once or twice a month on a consistent schedule. An effective strategy is to draft and schedule emails a month in advance; this will prevent scrambling at the last minute to put together an engaging email. Once patients get used to seeing your name pop up in their inboxes on a regular basis, they'll begin to expect your messages.

Customize Your Content

Avoid sharing cookie–cutter, templated materials. If you send the same emails as every other dentist on the block, you are not going to stand out. Email campaigns are a great way for your patients to get an idea of what makes your practice unique. Sharing things such as who you are, what you're about and what you appreciate about your patients will make them feel connected, and connectedness leads to loyalty. Loyal patients likely will not abandon you when a more conveniently located practice opens up, and they are more likely to refer you to their friends and family.

Track the Success of Your Emails

Another benefit of using email campaigns is that you can easily track their efficacy. You'll know if your subject lines are appealing by tracking how many recipients opened your email. You'll know your appointment request option is effective when a patient who hasn't been to your office in over a year clicks the "schedule an appointment" button. You can even find out how many people click the "read more" link after the content tease. If you send an informational email to 20 patients who have inquired about implants vs. dentures and eight of them call to schedule the procedures, you'll know that it was your email that gave them the extra encouragement they needed to follow through with pursuing treatment.

The most effective way to market your practice is to use a holistic approach. An inviting website and strong social media presence, combined with the strategic use of email, are the best ways to ensure that you are reaching your patients via multiple platforms.

This article originally appeared in the August/2016 issue of the Academy of General Dentistry's AGD Impact magazine.

The Strategy

Our goals are to enhance your business efforts beyond the doors of your practice and engage your patients more frequently than the two or three times a year that you see them for cleanings and checkups. As you know, some patients need more of a push to move forward with a service that they deem optional; additional education, an incentive, or simply a reminder to move forward may encourage them to follow through with a proposed treatment plan. In this case, we asked our client to identify the patients who had received consultations for Adult Orthodontics but had not pursued treatment.

With that information, we created a laser-focused promotional campaign. We used the email addresses of the clients who had been identified and sent a personal message to each, reminding them about their consultation for this treatment and offering an incentive to make their move. The offer, which ran for a limited time in June through August, was for $1000 off an Adult Orthodontic treatment. Once the emails were sent, we were able to track who opened the emails, who clicked on links to learn more, and who clicked the button to schedule an appointment. With this information, we were able to track the effectiveness of the campaign and use the data to optimize future strategies.

The Results

This simple strategy landed phenomenal results:

41 patients were contacted during a **3 month-long** campaign.

2 emails were sent to remind them of their treatment.

5 patients accepted treatment and scheduled an appointment for their Adult Orthodontic cases.

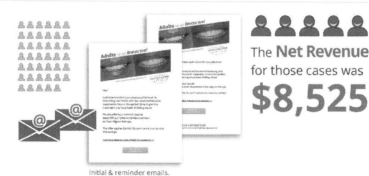

The **Net Revenue** for those cases was

$8,525

Initial & reminder emails.

CHAPTER THIRTEEN
An Effective Practice Website Is Key to Marketing Success

Dentistry is a highly competitive field. Modern dentists are making significant investments in technology and staff to differentiate themselves from their peers. Although your practice reflects your commitment to provide your patients with the best possible dental experience, another investment could be just as important to the future financial health and prosperity of your business—your practice's website.

More than one-third of your potential patients judge you based on the quality of your website, according to Futuredontics, the parent company of 1–800–DENTIST. First impressions can last forever, and they can determine whether or not a prospective patient decides to visit your practice or someone else's. So how does your website *really* look? There are key elements that every website should have to assure both its effectiveness and ease of use.

Selecting the Right Website Platform

There are a multitude of platforms available to create a website, and their effectiveness can vary greatly. There is the "Doc-in–the-box," or prepackaged solutions. These sites offer a menu of pre-categorized content to choose from, including images and features. However, they are based entirely on their perception (not yours) of your professional needs as a dentist. The copy is pre-written and not customized for your practice, and they usually feature stock photography.

Prepackaged solutions appear to be easy and cost-effective options, but, unfortunately, they lack originality and can have a noticeably negative impact on your Internet marketing strategy, minimizing its effectiveness. Search engines such as Google and Bing want to see original, easy-to-understand copy on your website, which helps improve your ranking in search results, and this "Doc-in-the-Box" option does not offer that.

If you are tech savvy, there are always do-it-yourself options. Multiple website building solutions allow you to easily plug in information and images into predesigned templates. Examples of these include Wix and GoDaddy website builder solutions. This do-it-yourself option is also cost-effective; however, building the actual site can be time-consuming, and they are usually not search engine optimization (SEO)-friendly.

WordPress is one publishing platform that is a viable option if you are building your own website. It gives you the ability to choose from an abundance of add-ons and themes to customize your website in a way that meets your specific needs. Without any required program knowledge, it also allows you to easily update your own website.

Whatever your final choice, you have to be sure the platform you use allows you to create a site that meets the needs of your practice, helps convert your visitors into patients, and gives you a solid foundation upon which to build your marketing activities. It also needs to be user–friendly and responsive on all devices (such as a desktop, laptop, tablet, and smartphone). Websites that are nonresponsive, or not mobile friendly, will appear lower in search results.

In early 2015, Google updated its search algorithm so that comparable mobile sites would rank higher than non–mobile friendly sites in mobile search results. This updated algorithm pushed all nonresponsive websites to the bottom of the search rankings.

According to Search Engine Land's "*Local Consumer Review Survey (2012),*" 85% of consumers use the Internet to search for local businesses, and more than 60% of Internet searches are done from a smartphone, according to Futuredontics. Not having a mobile–friendly website would be a waste of resources for your practice.

Attracting Prospective Patients with the Right Content

Content is one of the most important elements, if not the most important element, of your website—everything from the words on each page to the visuals you decide to use. Like the writer who has a sentence or a paragraph to get and keep his or her readers' attention, you will have mere seconds to stimulate a website visitor.

To be effective, the copy on your website must not only be fresh, interesting, and well–written, but also pertinent and beneficial to your website visitors. Why should they choose you as their dentist? Your website should clearly answer this question.

Although imitation is said to be the sincerest form of flattery, on the Internet it can lead to redundancy and result in lost interest among your website visitors and potential patients. Google is the largest and most widely used search engine in the world. It can recognize "canned content"—content that is generic or not written specifically for your practice—in an instant, deemphasizing or eliminating the site from search results and penalizing any organic targeted search for your dental services. If you are publishing content that is duplicated on hundreds, if not thousands, of other dental practice websites, you hurt your chances of prospective patients finding you. (These websites are also vying for the same dental–related traffic. There are more than 25,000 searches for dentists in Tampa, Florida, alone—imagine how many are searching in your area!)

Original dental website content that is updated often and search engine optimized will help your website stand out from your competition.

Enhancing the Esthetics of Your Website

Esthetics are another "make or break" aspect of your website. Don't overlook it. Use eye-catching and aesthetically pleasing colors and images to catch your visitors' attention. Take the time to personalize your site, injecting into it your personality and that of your staff. Your website is the outlet that should showcase how fun, friendly, cutting-edge, and welcoming your practice is and what your new patients can expect upon their first visit to your office. Patients want to see the real you. Use real images of your practice instead of stock photos. Tell those special, endearing stories of your patients' successes. Highlight information about the technologies your practice uses that will make a dental experience more enjoyable. Do you have an intraoral scanner that reduces time in the chair, eliminating the old "gunky" tasting impression material? Tell prospective patients about it in simple, easy-to-understand language. Do you offer weekend or evening appointments? Let them know! Why are you different from your competitors? This is the ideal forum to show that difference. Put your best dental foot forward. Be creative. Since we live in a social society, take advantage of it. Be sure that you have links to your social media accounts (such as Facebook, Twitter, and Instagram) that you are active on and that your patients are likely to frequent. If you don't stay relevant and meet them where they are, you can be sure that your competition will. In today's digitally evolving world, having an effective website is the first step to building a strong online presence. Your website should be the foundation of your marketing—one of your most economically feasible and effective tools to spread the word about your practice. Yet, it shouldn't be by chance. Take the time to regularly assess the effectiveness of your site. If you don't have one, make it your top priority. When potential patients are looking for you online, they need to be able to find exactly what you want them to see.

7 Things Your Dental Practice Website Must Have in 2016

- Responsive web design

- Clear and easy–to–understand page navigation

- Real images of you, your staff, and the office environment

- An easy-to-find call to action on the homepage, such as an appointment-request button or any new patient offers

- Links to your practice's social media accounts (Facebook, Twitter, Instagram

- Staff and doctor headshots with brief biographies

- Contact webpage with your office's phone number and address, as well as an inquiry form

This article originally appeared in the August/2016 issue of the Academy of General Dentistry's AGD Impact magazine

CHAPTER FOURTEEN
The Benefits of Blogging on Your Practice Website

"I'm a dentist. Why do I need a website or Facebook page? And if I have one, why do I still need a blog?"

How you react to these questions can impact the effectiveness of your marketing efforts and, ultimately, the profitability of your practice. We live in the Information Age, where your Internet presence can be just as important as the physical location of your practice and where potential patients can find you within seconds. And when they do find you, you should want them to see a consistent social media presence, a strong, organized website and, potentially, an up-to-date blog.

Benefits of Launching a Blog

Being relevant to current and prospective patients is an ongoing process. Since most of them will research you and your practice online before even making an appointment, what they see while they are searching should reflect your practice in the best possible light.

A blog is an important element of your website because it serves many purposes. Not only does it establish the dental expertise of you and your staff and position you as a thought leader, it also builds trust and credibility with your patients and increases your Internet visibility and brand awareness. Your blog is your public forum, and it provides the ideal opportunity to offer advice and tips to patients on their oral health.

When launching a blog, it is important that you house it on your own website, not on a separate site. If you're not sure how best to do that we'd highly recommend reaching out to your web developer for some assistance. It's usually very easy (and inexpensive) for a professional to add a blog to most websites. It does nothing to improve your practice website's ranking or searchability if it is hosted on another platform. Keep in mind that constantly updating your blog and, in turn, your website, with fresh content improves your search engine optimization (and, thus, your Google ranking), increases the potential for growing your site visitors (because they know you have up-to-date, quality information) and helps give you a leg up on your competition. A stale site and an unchanged, boring blog repels—as opposed to attracts—patients, defeating the purpose of blogging in the first place. Make your blog an ongoing part of the maintenance of your practice website.

Even with all of these benefits, your blog may not necessarily be an instant success in attracting new patients. It takes time to build a following, but eventually, the blog will help increase the awareness of your practice, its services, and other dentistry–related information. So don't be discouraged if your blog doesn't take off immediately. Continue to be consistent in offering blog content.

Blogging Best Practices and Tips

Let's look at your actual blog and the possibilities it affords. Follow the "KISS" rule, and keep it simple—from the look and layout of the blog to the language you use in each post. At the same time, blog posts should be interesting and relatable, and the language that you use in your blog posts should be easy for Google to understand. Yes, Google. The search engine considers both readability and the users' experience and determines how effective a Google search will be in reaching your website. One part of this is using keywords. Without doing in–depth keyword research, we'd suggest using keywords such as "dentist", "dentist <your city>", "dentist <your city>, <your state>", etc. These are likely the most popular keywords being searched in your region. Keywords are essential to searchability on particular topics, but adding words without purpose or overstuffing your blog with these key terms decreases your ranking with search engines and makes your site look like spam. The most effective method of implementing keywords into your text is to write intelligently and with the reader in mind.

Because your blog is an effective marketing tool, its visibility is of paramount importance. Share it with others. Post it on your practice's social media pages, or make it part of your monthly email campaigns. The greater the exposure, the greater the likelihood the reader will seek the source: your website.

Control the length of your blog posts. Try to write at least 300 words each time you blog. More would be better, but don't get verbose—your blog is not the place for your first novel. Too many words can turn off your readers just as easily as too few, encouraging them to find more interesting sites that offer engaging information that also can be easily digested. Examples of topics you could write about include: the benefits of dental implants (if that's a service you provide), how to determine if your patient is a candidate for veneers or other dental procedures, or dental prevention and the big picture. Talk with your patients, and find out what interests them. Or another good place to start is by considering some of the common questions patients ask you and your staff members.

We know how busy people are and the likelihood is that they will skim your blog, so make it easy for them to gain the important nuggets of information quickly. Use visuals, bullet and numbered lists, and bold subtitles that will allow them to scan your blog and maintain their attention.

And while you are doing that, don't make it dry. Put your personality into the blog. Make it personal, and don't forget your call to action. Tell them what you want them to do (for example, access a resource that's provided on your website). Don't assume they already know what your call to action is.

How often you blog is also important. Once a month is recommended as a minimum, but the more often you can do it, the better. At least once a week would be optimal.

If you lack either the time or ability to write an effective blog post, hire a dental marketing professional or agency that can help make your blog a powerful part of your marketing efforts.

This article originally appeared in the August/2016 issue of the Academy of General Dentistry's AGD Impact magazine.

CHAPTER FIFTEEN
Managing the Reputation of Your Dental Practice

Sally is a typical 21st century girl—wired up, logged in. Before a date, she Googles her suitor. Before going on vacation, she hits up TripAdvisor to size up her sleeping and dining options. But now Sally needs some dental work done. So what does she do?

She hits Yelp, Healthgrade, ZocDoc, and other review sites, checking out what patients of local practices have to say. Many local practices have no reviews, though. This doesn't pique her interest. She keeps scrolling. A few have patently bad reviews. Were these experiences perhaps rare exceptions at otherwise wonderful practices? She has no way of knowing. The pleased patients never left a review. So she scrolls some more.

Finally, she lands upon a practice, one of the few in the area with a robust bank of reviews, the overwhelming majority of them positive and garnering a full five stars. (Sure, there may have been one or two negative ones. But the sheer magnitude of positive reviews far outweighed them, in both the rating system and in Sally's assessment.) She's pleased with what she sees and makes her appointment.

After getting her dental work done, she's given simple instructions by the receptionist of the practice with a bit of motivation to leave a review herself. So she does, eager to share her pleasant experience with the rest of the world and adding to the practice's dazzling online reputation. And thus the cycle continues.

Manage Your Online Reputation

Sally is no outlier in terms of how she makes her choices. She represents the 90% of consumers who say online reviews influence their buying decisions. While word–of–mouth is a great means of advancing your name, in the age of information, nothing beats the ease with which we can Google a business and read what others have had to say about it in mere seconds. And this is rapidly changing how dental patients choose a practice.

In the past, it may have been normal to base choices simply on referrals, the doctor's credentials, and location. But today, it's referrals, location, and Internet presence. And, in addition to a sleek website, your online reviews constitute a major part of that presence. Moreover, because reviews increase new patients' trust, the more positive reviews you've got going on, the more trust they'll have.

But that reputation isn't going to happen by itself, is it? Too often, people are only compelled to leave reviews without outside prompting when their experience has been negative. As we saw with Sally, this can be a problem. This is why having a plan in place to obtain reviews from satisfied patients is absolutely essential. We prefer the "COME ON!" approach, which can be summed up as:

- Consistency in asking for reviews

- Office signage motivating patients to leave reviews

- Making it easy for your patients to leave reviews

- Email and marketing campaigns asking for reviews

- Ongoing monitoring and moderation of reviews

- Never leaving a negative review un–addressed

There's also an added side benefit of online reviews and citations: They boost your local SEO. This not only enhances your online reputation, but also your visibility. Online reputation management for dental practices has never been more important.

NOW IS THE TIME TO ACT

Finding exactly the right partner to move ahead can be a daunting challenge.

Anyone who tells you what to do without knowing who you are, what you are doing now, and where you want to end up in the future is at best misleading you (and at worst, lying to you).

A partner who takes you down this path with your marketing efforts could not only prove expensive, it very well could result in confused patients, diminishing case acceptance, and ruin your profitability and growth potential.

But there's another option—a simple first step that focuses on establishing a custom, personalized marketing strategy based on your own unique needs as a practice, doctor, team, and patient base. We call it:

"Your Practice Breakthrough Session"

What makes this step so powerful is the fact that you walk away with a marketing strategy 100% customized around the unique personality traits of YOUR practice and how others perceive it.

It involves a quick 30–minute call, is completely low stress, and requires zero upfront effort. All you need to do is dial. (*And we guarantee you'll be glad you did!*)

"Your Practice Breakthrough Session" will root out and identify in your practice any places where you're either making (or in danger of making) the five mistakes we've spoken about earlier. In addition, it examines the degree to which you're leveraging the "3Rs" in your practice—uncovering hidden "pain points" in your marketing strategy currently blocking new patients from walking in your door and potentially causing long-term patients to disappear forever.

So let's get into some specifics about what you can expect during **"Your Practice Breakthrough Session"...**

- First, it's DEFINITELY NOT about that tired, outdated "Marketing Plan" gathering dust on top of some office file cabinet. We're now in the "AGE OF AGILE"—where speed, focus, and action are critical to success—which is why you need to be able to BREAK THROUGH and move quickly in a way totally consistent your own unique Character and Purpose.

- Second, during our call we will together review your current online strategy to uncover untapped points of leverage and identify the best ways to structure your ongoing communication outreach to both New and Current Patients.

- Third, even though this session has a real-world value of $397, it's absolutely FREE. We're making it available as a gift to you just because you read this book—and being generous with our friends is just how we roll.

Spots are limited, however, so if you'd like to see your waiting room packed with new and returning patients, then act now to reserve your free **"Your Practice Breakthrough Session"** today by going to **PracticeBreakthroughSession.com.**

54723159R00059

Made in the USA
Columbia, SC
06 April 2019